I Dealt With Cancer and Won

(and kept it in remission for the past 26 years)

A True Story

by

Maxine Jannette

with

Julie C. Eger

I dealt with cancer and won/ Maxine Jannette - 1st Edition

ISBN -13: 978-1537184555 (pb)
ISBN -10: 1537184555
  1. Healthy Living - nonfiction
  2. Cancer - nonfiction

Cover Design by Maxine Jannette and Julie C. Eger

Dedicated to:

The rest of my life…

and

Anyone who is serious about dealing with cancer
in a more natural and holistic way.

Your body will thank you.

DISCLAIMER

This book is informational only and should not be considered as a substitute for consultation with a duly-licensed medical professional. Any attempt to diagnose and treat an illness should come under the direction of a physician. The author is not herself a medical doctor and does not purport to offer medical advice, make diagnoses, prescribe remedies for specific medical conditions or substitute for medical consultation.

While this story is true to the best of the author's knowledge, some names, businesses, and locations have been changed or shortened to protect the identities of the persons/places described.

TABLE OF CONTENTS

God hath not given us the spirit of fear; but of power, and love, and of sound mind.

2 TIMOTHY 1:7

Introduction

My name is Maxine. Most people have called me Mac, ever since I was little. But here's the thing that got me to thinking and 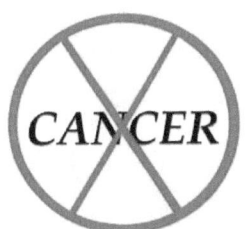 for a long time, it didn't make sense. When I was young, I had a friend. I met her in 1948 at the free picture shows they held over in Andalusia, Illinois. When my friend was ten-years-old she got leukemia. Then she died. From that time on, I always had a fear of getting cancer. I carried that fear for many years. It was instilled in me and seemed that it had to happen to me because I believed it would happen. I had accepted it. Those were my thoughts all those years.

Now, is it true? Because I had bought into the fear of getting cancer like my little friend did, is that why I got cancer? Did I bring cancer on myself or did it just fall out of the sky and land on me randomly, through no fault of my own? Is there something I could have done differently? Could I have eaten better? Could I have alleviated all the stress in my life more effectively? Did I really set the foundation for cancer to grow in me? Those are questions each cancer patient has to answer for themselves. And really, is there a correct answer? One that makes sense to all the people who have ever had any type of cancer?

Personally, I believe *my* thoughts about cancer had a lot to do with how cancer showed up in *my* life. But here's the thing. If my thoughts had that kind of power to invite cancer into my life, did my thoughts have the power to dismiss it as well? I didn't know if any of this made sense until I was faced with some tough decisions to make. This is my story and what I did when life, for whatever reason, dealt me the cancer hand. I made the decision to work on deleting the *thought* of cancer from my life and concentrate on other things. I made the decision to stop fearing cancer and that's when the shift began. This is how I played that hand.

February 1990

I had just turned 50 and I was starting to think I knew what it was.

The day I decided I had to do something about it, I was roofing. My husband, Jim, built houses for a living, and sometimes he had a small crew. I was always happy to step in and help. I loved the feel of wood in my hands. The feel of a hammer and nails. For whatever reason, I loved pounding nails the old-fashioned way, unlike the way they do nowadays. With those pneumatic nail guns. I liked pounding nails so much I entered a contest once. At Kindt Building Supply in Greenville, Wisconsin. A hammer and nail contest for women. I won first place. I took home a trophy and a $50 check as proof. Those are the kinds of things I was used to doing on a daily basis.

> I was always active in my life with gardening, taking care of grandchildren, and helping my husband build houses.

I was always active in my life with gardening, taking care of grandchildren, and helping my husband build houses. But during the month of February in 1990 I hadn't been feeling well. I thought it was something that would just go away. But it lingered. I didn't have any energy and that was so unlike me. I also noticed my skin was turning a sort of yellowish color. There was no oomph to my typical bounce.

Then one day in the middle of February we had to get Ted Rychtanek's roof on his new house because the guys putting up the drywall said they were coming. When the guys who did the drywall said they could come, everybody on the job jumped. If you missed the scheduled date for the drywall guys to come you never knew when they would be able to get back to the job. It could hold up work on a new house for weeks. And Ted Rychtanek was such a nice man we didn't want to make him wait.

The day in question was a very cold day, but that was okay. I was used to working in the cold. I had spent many hours mucking out pig and chicken pens in the cold during my teen years on my family's farm in Almond, Wisconsin. I had also spent many hours riding around a field on a tractor in 90°+ weather. The harsh elements handed out by Mother Nature were a normal part of my life. I didn't question it. I learned to adapt to it.

While working on Ted's new house, my job was to get the shingles on the roof. My husband set me up with two guys to work with. I was working on the north side of the new house. The two hired helpers worked on the south side of the house so they were out of the wind. You see, I didn't like to put other people in the worst type of situation. I would rather deal with the worst myself. It wasn't a matter of thinking about it one way or the other. That's just how I was raised. In my family it was an unwritten rule to give the best to others first. No questions asked. In the long run, I think it made me a strong person. Anyway…

That day it was just below zero degrees. It was a bone chilling kind of cold. I worked straight through until I got my side of the roof done. But by the end of the day I felt just terrible. I was so sick. I was so weak. But I did it. I finished putting on that roof with my Pa's words ringing in the back of my head..."You've got to finish this job with no complaints." It was how he was raised and it was how he raised me.

But the next day I called a clinic down in the southeastern part of the state. It was rare for me to go see a doctor. But this felt like something bigger than a lingering sore throat, bronchitis or some odd kind of stomach flu. I had handled those things on my own for the better part of my life. So I made the appointment, February 15th, a Thursday. I thought it was my good fortune they were able to squeeze me in.

Once the nurses got me all checked in and took my vitals I got to meet the doctor. I told him what I was experiencing. Then they took some tests. Blood tests. Urine test. Poking around in unmentionable parts of my body for *samples*. Right there in the examining room. Back then it wasn't like it is today. Now you go through a lot of tests with a lot of specialists, but back then everything happened in one small examining room.

I waited about three hours and then the doctor walked back into the room with a grave look on his face.

Grave.

Grave is not the kind of look you want to get from your doctor.

Grave is not the kind of look you want to get from your doctor. A grave is too closely connected to *death*. I waited to hear what he had to say. And then he said the word everyone dreads.

Something...something...blah...blah...blah... cancer of the breast, liver and bowel. And then he said the other words no one wants to hear. "With the type of cancer you have, you probably have six months to live. We can maybe extend the time to ten months if you immediately have surgery on your liver."

> *"Possibly with surgery on my liver, I might have ten months to live?"*

This thought pinged around inside my skull like one of those little balls in a pinball machine. Ping! Ping! Ping!

In a daze I heard someone saying they ought to go soak their heads. Someone was saying, "If this is all the time you're giving me, well then, I guess I'll be just fine." It turned out that *someone* was *me* talking. I still have a hard time believing I would talk to a doctor that way. So disrespectful. I was taught that even if you didn't like what someone had to say you didn't sass them back. But this odd, fuzzy conversation continued on. A nurse was telling me I should call my family and get my affairs in order. That I would have to sign papers saying I would agree to have surgery on my liver.

In a blur, the nurse had the papers ready, sitting on the counter. I picked up the pen. I could feel that pen in my hand. The nurse turned to do something. She stood with her back to me. The papers were there and it was like a huge pendulum was nudging me, but I couldn't get that pen to sign the papers. It was like signing my death certificate and I just couldn't do that. I decided right then and there I was going to have to do this a different way, even though at the time I wasn't sure what that way was going to be. I put the pen down and walked out of the office.

When I left the clinic, after they told me I might have only six months to live, as I was coming up Highway 41, I started crying. I thought, "Oh crap." So I pulled over and I'm sitting there crying and finally I said, "Okay, dummy. You can fix this. You don't need this kind of stuff bothering you in your life." I stopped crying, dried my tears and drove home. My goal was to find answers. The search was on.

When I got home I told my husband a doctor told me I had cancer. My husband looked at me for a long moment and said, "We'll get through this." My gut feeling was he didn't believe anything in our life would change. We had a habit of keeping to ourselves, so neither one of us told anyone. I hate to bother people with my problems, so it was easier to just not say anything. I'm like an old dog that will crawl under the porch to heal when I don't feel well. Stay there in the quiet and lick my wounds until they're gone. I think I was already thinking I didn't want to bring attention to this. That it was important to head into that place under the porch. That somehow, attention would make this cancer thing bigger. I couldn't handle anything much bigger than this. But that was just an inkling of a thought at the time. I didn't realize until later how important this thought was going to be.

> But that was just an inkling of a thought at the time. I didn't realize until later how important this thought was going to be.

For the next couple of weeks, the doctor's office called me every day. They might have missed a couple of days. But they were calling all the time. Telling me I should get in there and start getting something done with chemo and radiation, whatever. I had thought that particular clinic was more natural than other clinics, as there was beginning to be a trend toward more natural ways of healing at that time.

> I finally told my husband, the next time they call just tell them I died so they'll leave me alone.

I guess I was wrong about that. It seemed the nurses were calling all the time. I finally told my husband, the next time they call just tell them I died so they'll leave me alone. At that time, I was so depressed I went to Carter's Photography Studio in Berlin, Wisconsin and had him take a professional photo of me. Even though I hated having my picture taken. In case I died. So my family would have something to remember me by. It was one of the saddest days of my life. Sometimes, to this day, I search my eyes in those photographs, trying to see if I pulled it off. If happiness was evident in my eyes, or did the sadness show through enough for folks to see I was faking it. Because at that point, I was scared senseless.

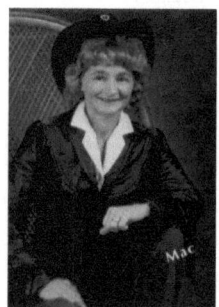 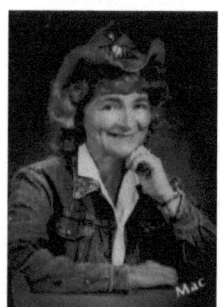

It was interesting that soon after I told my husband what to tell the nurses the next time they called from the doctor's office, they stopped calling. Just like that. My husband never did get a chance to tell them I died. Which is probably a good thing because it wasn't true. I was just so tired of them calling and harassing me all the time. At least it felt like harassing to me, even though I know they believed they were trying to help. I was so tired of them putting all that on me when I'd made my decision to do things, as Frank Sinatra so elegantly sang it, *my way*. And I was only beginning to figure out what *my* way was.

March 1990

We were still living on the hill just off of Hwy F near Silver Lake in Wautoma. Jim was running his construction business. I would help when I could. Things were crazy around our house like they'd been ever since he started his business. Back then we didn't have cell phones. Our phone rang off the hook every morning and evening with people calling trying to catch Jim before he headed out to work or as soon as he got home at night.

I had made the decision to keep the news about me having cancer to myself. I was still tied to the idea where the old dog crawled under the porch so it could heal. A big part of me didn't want to interrupt anyone else's life because of what was going on with me. I didn't want to worry anyone. It never crossed my mind to tell other folks because *they* might care about *me*. I was pretty independent and I thought I was good at taking care of myself and everybody else, too.

At that point, my husband was the only one who knew about the doctor's diagnosis but I did finally mention it to my mother. I still hadn't said anything to my children. Before I said too much, I wanted to know, really, what I was talking about. This was all new to me. I needed time to do some research, get my hands on a book or some information about people who had survived a diagnosis such as mine. Back then we didn't have computers and the internet to find information. We had to rely on the local library, catalogs, magazines, and printed out books. Or you had to know somebody who knew somebody who knew somebody who had gone through a successful treatment for the kinds of cancer I had. That meant asking around for help. I was concerned if I asked too many questions, someone would figure out what was going on with me, and I wasn't ready for that.

But it was interesting what happened after I told my mother. I will say that what happened will not be true for some people, but it turned out to be true for me. When I told my mother, the first thing she said was, "I'm going to put you on the prayer chain at church." I thought that was a good idea.

> But then things took a bad turn.

But then things took a bad turn. I began to feel worse. In my mind I was making the connection with the prayer chain at church, and a thought jumped into my head one day. It stopped me right in my tracks.

Someone isn't praying right.

> *"Someone isn't praying right."*

I wasn't sure what that meant at the time, but I knew the thought that jumped into my head was important. Very important. I began to understand it had something to do with focusing on the negative. Someone was putting huge amounts of focus on what was going wrong instead of what could go right. It was one of those things, that at the time, I didn't know would turn out to be important for me in the long run. Not just with what someone else was thinking and how they were thinking about the cancer, but how *I* was thinking about the cancer. I called my mother and told her to immediately take me off the prayer chain. I don't know what she told them but they stopped. It wasn't long, and things began to turn around again. I was still not well, but at least I wasn't feeling worse.

For years, since back in the 1960s, I'd been drawn to things natural and organic. Back then I was accused of being organic before being organic was cool. But when I was young, we didn't call it organic food, we just called it food. But something inside me always believed the doctors had been missing a very important aspect of health. I believed food was medicine, and medicine should be able to be used as food, interchangeably.

I understood the theory of having to stay on a regulated amount of medicine for a certain amount of time when it came to prescriptions. Then when you were well enough you would have to go off the prescription medicine. Staying on the medicine for too long, especially some of the stronger medications; would kill you. I was looking for something I could do for the rest of my life. However long that might be.

I had another belief that went against everything the doctors told me. Years before a friend of mine, Leroy Wruck, mentioned to me, "A man once told me that no matter what problem or illness you might have in your life, you must love *it*. Whatever *it* is." I wasn't sure I had heard him right, but I felt that what he shared was true, even though at the time, I couldn't exactly put my finger on why I believed it was true. He said I had to love it.

> He said I had to love it. So I mulled that over in my mind, trying to wrap my head around it.

So I mulled that over in my mind for awhile, trying to wrap my head around it. I figured it wouldn't cost anything to change my thinking, and I didn't have anything more to lose. I mean, they'd already told me I didn't have long to live. So, I went about changing my mind, changing my thoughts. And it was strange. I really did start to feel better. A little.

Then I had a revelation. I remembered my little friend who had died of leukemia when she was only ten-years-old. And how afraid I'd been all my life that someday something like that might happen to me. And then someday came. The diagnosis of cancer. Of the liver, the breast and the bowel.

> "That fateful day is the day I had a revelation that rocked my world."

The fear, it was right there. I was carrying that fear all that time since I was ten-years-old. I was carrying around the idea that cancer was a scary thing. I began to realize I had to do what I could to make it so cancer wasn't so scary. That it was manageable. That a person could beat it. Overcome it. Maybe even, *embrace* it. In other words, *love it,* just as Leroy's friend had said to do. Maybe there was something I could do to make it seem as though the cancer wasn't so scary. All I had to go on was what I had previously heard about cancer. But maybe everything I'd heard wasn't necessarily true. Maybe, *just maybe,* cancer wasn't as scary as everyone had led me to believe.

I made a conscious decision. I took responsibility for my thoughts as soon as I realized what I had been doing, about how I had been thinking. For the first time I could remember, when I thought about cancer I decided I wasn't going to be afraid. If I thought about it at all, I was going to think about it with a big X running through it, as though it didn't even exist. To cancel it out. I would cancel out cancer. But would that work? Could I just *pretend* the cancer away? And if so, how would I go about doing that?

I knew the cancer was there. They said it was. Those doctors. They had tests to prove it. I understood that just pretending it wasn't there wasn't going to make it go away. But neither was fighting with it. At that point I had all these little voices inside my head telling me what I should do and what I shouldn't do. I began to notice how critical those niggling little thoughts were. Negative little thoughts. Never-ending little thoughts. Tormenting little thoughts. Demon-like. It was like a cartoon I'd seen once with a devil on one shoulder and an angel on the other. There was a devil on one shoulder trying to overpower the angel on my other shoulder. He was sitting there and he wouldn't shut up. But even if he was talking, talking, talking, did I have to listen to what he had to say about the doom and destruction of my body?

I began to understand I needed to begin a new conversation inside myself and I needed to do it fast. I needed to start up a conversation with that little angel and only listen to *that* voice. The devil could do what he wanted, but then, so could I. So I began to define things more as to what I wanted. This I knew. I wanted the devil to shut up, because he was driving me crazy with all that negative talk inside my head, but he wouldn't be quiet. And I didn't know how to make him shut up. What was making him so powerful, yakking in my ear all the time with his negative thoughts? Where was he getting all this power from? Was I doing something to make him stronger? Was I supposed to shift my thinking in order to cancel out his constant negative chatter? So that even if he kept on talking, talking, talking I wouldn't be able to hear him? What would it take for that to happen? What did I want more than anything? Then it hit me. Did I even know what I really wanted? Maybe that was the place to start. I had to define even more specifically what I wanted more than anything.

So I made a decision and became clearer in my thinking. This is what I wanted. I simply wanted the cancer to go away and not hurt anybody. I didn't want it to have the power to hurt me or anybody else. Something inside me clicked that it was the simplicity of my true desire that was a big part of the solution. Then it occurred to me the cure for this dilemma could be just as simple.

I also remembered something my mother had once said to me, "The devil *loves* a good fight."

> "The devil *loves* a good fight."

It was an old saying, but it seemed valid, based on what I was experiencing. I started to realize that if I was fighting with the devil it would only make him stronger and happier. And that would leave me powerless and unhappy. The light bulb went on above my head, big time.

> *"That's what Leroy's friend meant when he said you have to love it!"*

I wasn't supposed to fight the cancer because the negativity of the fight made the devil stronger. It made the cancer stronger. The most effective way to fight the devil, to fight the cancer, was with *love*. But then the question switched to; how exactly, was I supposed to do that?

I started to realize I was having a hard time concentrating and in order to change my thoughts and stop listening to the constant negative chatter inside my head I had to be able to concentrate. I had to be able to focus.

For years our life had been like Grand Central Station. People coming and going, phone ringing all the time. I was crazy busy with all the accounting work I did to keep track of what was going on with our construction business. I'd like to point out that, in my opinion, having your own business is a lot different than having a job where you punch in at 9:00 and punch out at 5:00. It isn't the kind of job where you can go home and forget about everything that happened at work and leave it for your boss or manager to worry about. When you have your own business, you are at the mercy of other people, and any of those people have the potential to become your *temporary* employer. They could be the one person who writes your paycheck for the next month, so you try to be nice to everybody, just in case they turn out to be your temporary employer.

It's a tricky balancing act when you're trying to please any one who might become your employer. Sometimes if you take time off for yourself you might step on one of your potential employer's toes and they'll become frustrated or impatient and go hire someone else. We worked hard to try and make everyone happy. It was part of our work ethic, plus we had bills to pay. But it was also exhausting trying to please so many people.

It seemed like a frenzy of noise inside my head, all that racket, when I had this life or death situation to face.

The other thing that seemed to interfere with my ability to concentrate was my husband and the things he liked. He liked to watch TV and listen to the radio. It seemed like a frenzy of noise inside my head, all that racket, when I had this life or death situation to face. Sometimes I had the urge to throw a brick through the TV when everyone was laughing over make-believe situations portrayed on TV, whether they were crying over spilled milk, shooting a make-believe bad guy or blowing up make-believe cities while I was supposed to be fighting for my life.

And there was still the phone, always ringing. And then my husband was looking at some land he wanted to buy, a place where, if we moved there, we would have to build a house as the old house had burned down. It was an old farm-turned-hunting-resort near the Wautoma Airport. There were two big pole sheds and a smaller building; a string of rooms the last owner had used as an eight-room motel unit for duck hunters. The place needed a lot of work. And I was exhausted. I had no idea how we'd be able to pull off the repairs to those buildings, plus build a house, if our offer to purchase was accepted. But it was, so we became the owners of this *'new to us'* place. But in the back of my mind, it meant more money spent. And if I couldn't help with the work, where was the money supposed to come from? And what would happen if I racked up a bunch of hospital bills?

It was coming onto springtime and I found myself feeling sad. I never noticed when the robins came back, which was usually around the 10th of March. I had always been busy during the month before spring arrived, planning a big vegetable garden. But this year was the first year of my life I didn't think about my garden. I did everything except get ready to put in a garden. That alone told me my situation was serious.

It was a tug-of-war and I felt like I was losing.

And then I came across a book called *How to Fight Cancer & Win* by William L. Fischer. (available now on Amazon) I knew if I could just wrap my head around that kind of information I would be okay. I started to apply some of the things I read about in his book. But then I ran into a couple of snags.

April 1990

After a month of trying to live my life like I'd been used to living it, I realized I had to make a change or die. The way I was living was going to kill me; for two reasons I could see. I had what the doctor said was a killing kind of cancer. And it seemed impossible for me to think clearly and concentrate on what I could do to change this killing cancer with all the chaos going on around me *and* the chaos running rampant inside my own head. At least it felt like chaos, chatter on the inside, chatter on the outside. But even though I was having a hard time concentrating, one thought kept finding its way into my head. It was around this time I began to realize I had to stop calling it *my* cancer, and start calling it *the* cancer.

> If I bought into the fact it was *my* cancer, then I would own it.

If I bought into the fact it was *my* cancer, I would own it. Who wants to own cancer? The more I owned *it*, the more *it* had power over me. If I kept it distant, then the power it had over me might grow to be less and less. Somewhere inside me, I knew I had to be able to concentrate on what I could do to change the *killing cancer* situation. Instead of focusing on what the doctor said was a *killing cancer,* it occurred to me that maybe I could *kill* the cancer instead. With kindness. And with love, as my friend Leroy had suggested. More and more I began to get the gist of what Leroy and his friend had said.

I began to realize I needed a break from my life because the life I was living, the life I'd created, was going to kill me. It became apparent, I needed to change my life, and in order to do that, the first thing I could do to rectify this situation was to change *myself.* But first, I had to be able to focus and to do that I needed to leave my current life and start taking care of *me*.

I wasn't willing to put myself first in the beginning. My husband was used to depending on me to run and get supplies. I was good at getting supplies. But now I was sick and I was so tired. There was tension between us and I felt he wasn't able to understand what I needed to do to get well.

And then, there were my friends.

> I began to focus on removing negative things from my life. Some of the hardest negative things to remove were...people.

I began to focus on removing negative things from my life. Some of the hardest negative things to remove were...people. How would I remove them and feel good about my decision? I didn't want to be mean to them, but I didn't want to die either. I felt like I was suffocating under the weight of what other people would want me to do instead of what I wanted to do. Could I make them feel included if they were going to fight me? What would I say to those I knew would disagree with my decision? Especially the people I thought I loved, the ones I cared about. The people I had been in relationships with for a long time.

Some of my closer friends started to notice my lack of *participation* in things we normally did. They started to ask questions. The more they wanted to know, the more I pulled away. The more I pulled away, the more curious they became. And the more curious they became the more questions they'd ask. It was beginning to be a vicious cycle that was wearing me down. I knew I couldn't avoid them forever. A few of my friends started to suspect what was going on. They kept insisting I should go to the doctor and do whatever the doctor said. Now I had another thing to fight with. If I let them in on what was going on, I knew from past experiences, they would try to force me to do something I had already decided against. I knew what *they* thought about cancer. Some of them just wouldn't listen to what *I* had to say about doing things my way. And I was so tired. And I still hadn't told my children.

I wanted to immerse myself in William Fischer's book about how to beat cancer so I could develop a plan of action tailor-fit for me and my situation. I needed more time to do research and I felt like some people were backing me into a corner. I kept avoiding them so I could learn more about doing this naturally, but I was running out of time and energy. And I knew I couldn't keep hiding and keep my friends too. It came down to, which friends would support me and which friends wouldn't?

And then there was the financial aspect of the whole thing that kept popping up in the back of my mind. I began to realize worrying about money wasn't going to help me get well. How many times do we put our work before our own health because we think we need to make money to pay bills, especially big hospital bills or to make the payment on the insurance premium? At that time, we had no health insurance, so our worries were a bit different than those who did. If things got really bad, how in the world would we pay for this? But I had to put that kind of thinking aside. I needed to listen to what my body needed no matter what my financial situation was. No matter what other people thought they needed from me. And it was a hard decision on where to draw that line.

I drew the line. I tackled the problem with my husband first. It was true I needed to change. I told him I couldn't do it anymore, all the work I'd been doing. And get rid of the TV and radio constantly making noise in the background of my life. The never-ending drone of sound.

I told my husband, "If you want to be around me, I'd like for you to be positive." I got a strange look from him and knew that was going to be impossible for him to do at that point. I didn't need to say anything else. I had drawn a line and so had he. We were on opposite sides and I realized I was going to have to do much of this on my own. I was sad about the line, but I knew it would be easier in the long run if he kept his negativity to himself.

So I left my husband at the old house and I moved to the new place we'd bought, the place most people in Wautoma remember where they grew acres of strawberries over by the airport. I moved into the building that had been used as migrant housing before they turned it into a motel for duck hunters. I moved into rooms Number 1 and 2.

I took some clothes, my dog, and my chickens. I wasn't sure if it was the right thing to do, but I thought it would give me time and space to clear my mind so I could change my thinking, quiet the devil chattering in my head, and start learning how to love this cancer-thing enough to keep it from doing any more damage.

It was true I needed to change.

Those abandoned motel rooms were quiet. They were at the end of a dead end road overlooking a beautiful swamp. I could see the swamp from the south window in room Number 1. As the sandhill cranes and the geese settled in for the summer I began the process of learning to delete all the negative images of cancer I'd ever heard about. I had found a place where outside influences couldn't reach me. No telephones. No TV. No radio. I was in a place where I could practice focusing and thinking positively. I was in a place where I didn't have to fight with people or defend my decision about trying to do this my way. There was no one around to bother me. I had just my own self to take care of.

I left all the coming and going of work related things. I was fortunate I didn't have to quit a job I would never get back once I left. I know losing a job is a huge concern for many people when they receive news they are facing a serious illness. It's bad enough when you receive the news when you are retired but when you are still working and have a family to provide for, it can be extra devastating. I worked at home so of course that part suffered. But if I got well, I could always get that back. If I still wanted to go back to that kind of life. Which was another inkling of an idea. It was the first step in learning how I was going to do this thing. My way.

When I went to live at the motel, when I left my old life behind, it was interesting. The friends who didn't agree with my decision automatically weeded themselves out of my life. I didn't have to do anything. They made their choices, frustrated and disgusted with me and my seemingly-crazy choice, and they left. This included my husband. He knew he couldn't be the positive person I needed him to be, so he too, left me alone. He didn't leave forever, but he stayed away during that time. It was like a blessing in disguise. It wasn't that they didn't matter. It was just that we had each made a decision that took us in a different direction. It was a relief not to have to worry about fighting with them about my decision. It was a relief not to have to worry about what I would say to these people who knew about my choice. But there were still others out there who didn't know yet. I still needed to tell my kids. But I also needed to figure out what was keeping me from telling them. I had to identify the fear that was all tangled up with that. What was holding me back from sharing this news with them?

And still, I needed to feel safe so I could explore and I needed time so I could experiment with these kinds of things that weren't very popular back then. So I locked myself in the motel. Now I could concentrate on *me*.

But it was tough. This was brand new to me. Taking care of myself. At the time of the diagnosis, I was used to putting everyone else first. My family, friends, even strangers had always come first in my life before my own health. I had never thought about that before, that in choosing to take care of others first it could lead to a decline in *my* health. But I could see it then. After the diagnosis. They say hindsight is 20/20.

I was learning about where to draw the line when it came to my health. I could see that if I failed to take care of me first, then I wouldn't be able to help others. Inside me, I'd always felt driven to help others. My first recollection of what I wanted to be when I grew up was a doctor. I loved farming. I loved carpentry. But being a doctor…it seemed I could never get that out of my head. I'd always thought that would be a wonderful way to help people, if you did it right.

I felt that because I'd spent so many years dreaming about what it would be like to help others it took some major focusing to visualize myself at the *front* of that line. I had been taught to *never* put myself first. But I knew that had to change. It could be possible, but for me it had to include huge amounts of humility. The idea of being selfish or arrogant was not an option for me. It felt like it went against the grain of who I was, or even more so, who I believed I wanted to be.

I was spending time preparing my new home in those two motel rooms. Cleaning out cobwebs of old stuff. Dusting off things I'd never seen before. I thought of the implications of being on a dead end road and how that could seem like the *end*. But I realized it was exactly what I needed to put the old stuff behind. When one thing ends, another thing begins.

> When one thing ends, another thing begins.

I built something like a nest in those motel rooms. I'd listen closely before I opened the door to the outside, making sure no one was there before I stepped out. I strolled along the edge of the swamp, listening to the sounds of Mother Nature, noticing the colors and the beauty. Then I began to hear something else. It was the sound of a little voice inside me, sort of like *The Little Engine Who Could,* a story about a little train engine written by Watty Piper. And something began to shift.

May 1990

May burst open in the swamp. Red-winged blackbirds were having their second clutch of babies, the father bird driving away anything that came near the nest. Tch, tch, tch. Tch tch, tch. The remaining pair of sandhill cranes nesting in the swamp had two babies. I could see nests of barn swallows tucked in against the beams of the pole building and under the eaves of the motel. Mothers and babies everywhere. I was starting to relax. I was thinking more clearly. This move had been a good thing. It was working. Kind of. I was forming a plan where I would leave much of it to fate as far as my kids were concerned. And by *it,* I meant my *condition. The cancer.* But Mother's Day was right around the corner and I was starting to feel a bit melancholy, trying to pin down my feelings about what to say to my kids while trying to figure out what to do about my health.

I spent hours immersing myself in William Fischer's book about how to fight cancer. I was fascinated by the success stories of Dr. Ann Wigmore's wheatgrass therapy. There was a place in Wautoma where I could buy it. It was all the way on the other side of town but it was frozen. I was facing a life or death situation and I wanted to get the freshest wheatgrass possible, so I started growing my own. These days there are all kinds of places to get good wheatgrass if you just go online and look. It's a lot easier to get it now than it was back in the early '90s. But what I planted grew quite quickly so I had fresh wheatgrass pretty much right away.

It was about this time I started to pull from my experience of dealing with difficult weather all my life. Learning to deal with different types of weather all those years was a big help to me. I knew there was no way to change the weather, so I had to learn different ways to deal with it. I began to apply that kind of thinking so *I* could change. How could I adapt to this thing called cancer? What did I need to know that I didn't know? Who could I talk to who knew about cancer? I also began to change my eating habits tremendously. Lots of green stuff. Lots of vegetables. Poached fish. Raw nuts and seeds.

It wasn't until years later I realized one of the reasons I was able to beat the cancer was because the foods I had chosen were so alkaline. But so was positive thinking. I didn't realize it at the time, but I was alkalizing my body and I learned even later that cancer cannot exist in an alkaline environment. At least that's what I believe now. In my opinion, cancer could only survive where there is too much acid. (Possibly too much alkaline too, but that was not my case, and that is another story).

I also figured that fear itself is -- acidic. It's like anger. It gets hot in your body, like battery acid, and it will burn. So where there is fear, cancer can grow and thrive. When a doctor tells you that you only have six months to live, that's pretty darn scary. I think some people die right then, or at least the part of them that wants to live dies, right there on the spot because the fear changes something inside you so it feels like you are dead. But I learned to love the cancer. I learned to have no fear of it. I just loved it, and maybe it loved me back. I don't know. But I think loving it changed it so it couldn't do any harm. It wasn't cancer anymore, once I loved it so much. It was something like cancer at that point, but it also stopped being a cancer that could kill.

So I persevered.

I was making fresh carrot juice and fresh celery juice every day with the most organic foods I could get my hands on.

Back then I juiced most every organic raw vegetable I could get my hands on. It was a tough time of year as new foods hadn't begun to grow in the region where I lived, but I did buy carrots by the 25# bag from a food co-op. I went through a lot of carrots. And celery. I was making fresh carrot juice and fresh celery juice every day. Every morning I just used my regular blender to grind things up and make my juice. I'd drink it, pulp and all.

I started eating a mixture of foods suggested by Dr. Johanna Budwig in William Fischer's book about how to fight cancer. Dr. Budwig recommended a combination of essential fatty acids which can be found in linseed (flaxseed) oil and proteins (with sulfur as their base) which can be found in cottage cheese or yogurt. Dr. Budwig used cottage cheese but I used plain yogurt with flax oil, flax seeds, walnuts or almonds with a little bit of fruit added in (strawberries were my favorite) and a few drops of organic stevia. There was a picture of the recipe in the book of how to layer everything in with the cottage cheese, but I would just mix it in a blender until it was all ground up and very creamy. It was easy and quick to make. It was exceptionally good tasting, at least it was to me. In fact, it was so good I still eat it for my breakfast nearly every day. I'm a believer that if you find something that works, it makes good sense to stick with it.

I was doing all these things that were supposed to be good for me. But there was a little dark cloud hanging over me. Well, a dark cloud and a bright cloud. Sort of bittersweet. Mother's Day was getting closer and I knew I was going to have to spend time with my kids. I mean, I was glad I was still here on Mother's Day and I could be with my kids. *That* was the bright spot. It could have been very different. But I knew I had to tell my kids what was going on and Mother's Day had become D-Day for me. *That* was the dark spot. I was really struggling with how to handle the whole cancer thing when it came to my kids. I decided to give my children those professional photos I'd had taken back in February. I had the photos framed, wrapped them up and held my breath as my children opened them. I was waiting for the right moment to tell them the news about what the doctor had said. But when they saw the pictures of me that I'd given them, I knew they already knew.

I didn't know *how* they knew because I hadn't said anything yet. And no one else had said anything to them either. I had asked my mother, husband and friends to not say anything as I wanted to tell my children the news myself, in my own way. I believed everyone had kept their promise to let me tell my children in my own way, in my own time. But secretly, I was hoping I would get better, fast, so I would never have to say anything at all about the doctor's diagnosis.

But my daughters knew. I didn't find out until later how they knew, but my daughter said it best in a poem she wrote years later. It tells the story better than I can about how they figured it out without me saying anything. It tells how they felt about my decision. They were very upset. Upset because I had cancer. And upset because I hadn't told them sooner. I must admit there was a power struggle going on. I was glad I had the strength to say what *I* felt no matter how *they* felt. My daughters were a force to be reckoned with. They were strong young women on their own, but combined they were even stronger. When I told them what the doctor had said they were going to hog-tie me and drag me back to the doctor. That's how afraid they were. But I told them they would have to catch me first. That is, *if* they could find me. This whole scenario gives you a pretty good idea how we handled things in my family. There always seemed to be threats that involved someone being hog-tied or whacked upside the head with a two-by-four to knock some sense into their addled head.

Here is my daughter's poem that tells what happened on that day.

My Mother's Doves
By Julie C. Eger © 2010

We didn't know until
she gave us the pictures,
those professional photos of herself,
for Mother's Day,
this, the woman who could smell
a camera coming
she, who could duck behind a counter
quicker than anyone I knew in order
to dodge having her picture taken.
My sister and I figured it out.
Mother was dying, and this was
her way of telling us
because she wouldn't talk about death.
When we confronted her, she said
she'd made her decision four months ago
when they gave her six months to live.
No more cutting, she said.
I'm doing this my way,
and if you're not with me, you're against me
and I'm telling you right now, I would love
to have your support because I can't fight this
and the both of you. We all cried then.
Fifteen years later she told me
about the doves -
how she pictured them every day,
pecking away the little pieces
of cancer and carrying them
to a place where
they couldn't hurt her anymore,
where they couldn't hurt anyone else.
It was very important they drop the pieces
where they couldn't hurt anyone else.

(An earlier version of this poem appeared in:
Perennial - poems   that last… by Julie C. Eger - 2016)

After my daughters cornered me and wrestled the truth from my very defensive self, my daughters confronted me with the question, "Did it ever occur to you to give us a chance to support your decision and show you how much we cared?"

> "Did it ever occur to you to give us a chance to support your decision and show you how much we cared?"

I had been afraid they would fight me on my decision and it just seemed easier to go ahead and do what I was going to do, no matter what they said. But I must admit, once they knew, things got easier and I was glad they decided to support me. Wholeheartedly. Unabashedly. No matter how they truly felt.

I continued with the wheatgrass, the juicing, and Dr. Budwig's sulfur-based protein/essential fatty acid recipe. I chose to continue spending most of my time alone at the motel. My daughters would occasionally stop over to help with things I needed a hand with. They couldn't call because I had no phone. I knew being independent was a very important part of my healing process. Answering to someone else just wasn't in the cards for me. I knew if I needed help, all I had to do was ask. But asking went against the grain of my gut feeling. For whatever reason, I needed to figure this out on my own. Well, with God's help. By this time, God and I were a pretty good team.

I read everything I could get my hands on about people who survived cancer. I applied what they said. I talked to positive people. I followed their lead. I was still juicing most every organic raw vegetable I could get my hands on. I was still growing my own wheatgrass and putting it into my blender. I made a couple of fresh batches every day. In addition to all those things, I started to practice positive thinking.

I will say this. Maybe it wasn't what was in the nuts and seeds. Maybe it wasn't the juicing of all those carrots and celery and other vegetables. Maybe it wasn't the wheatgrass. Maybe it wasn't the linseed (flax) oil. Maybe it wasn't the positive thinking itself. What I think it was, was a combination of all those things put together that created the key for me to open the door to my own health.

> What I think it was, was a combination of all those things put together that created the key for me to open the door to my own health.

I believe the way I used all of those things together is what was effective for me. I don't believe medicine or health is a one-size-fits-all kind of thing. I think each person has to tinker with a few different things to find out what will work best for them. If you listen to your body you will see that it is always nudging you in the right direction.

I think the addition of the positive thinking I began to introduce is what pulled it all together for me. And having all those things work together in my favor is what began to pull me out of the belief the doctors nearly had me believing, that I was headed for the grave.

I worked hard on eliminating my fear of cancer, constantly going back in my head to redirect my thinking, rewire my brain. Leroy's friend had said to *love* it, but he never said anything about not fearing it. That one I came up with on my own, on a clear day, sitting there looking out over the swamp.

The thought just seemed to jump into my head. How fear was the opposite of love.

I said to myself, okay, I need to love this cancer. It's a part of me. And I came to love it, and I felt it with every fiber of my being; every inch of everything I am. I loved it. Once in awhile something negative would jump into my head, not always about the cancer, but other negative things; and I practiced deleting them. I began training myself to believe that love could conquer anything that showed up. Even cancer. I had read in a book (I wish I could remember the name of it, but alas, it escapes me. It was twenty-six years ago!) where this lady had cancer. She was surrounded by chaos and no matter how hard she tried to be alone, those peaceful, alone times were far and few in between. She had to wait until she had a chance to be alone. But when she was alone she would visualize a PacMan-like character gobbling up all the bad parts.

I began to visualize a little yellow-colored blob, kind of like the one in that *PacMan* game the kids used to play on video games. The yellow blob would gobble up all the cancer and drop it off in a place where it could do good things instead of bad things. And then I thought it would be a good idea to get those pieces even further away than that, so I started visualizing doves. White doves. Dozens of them. They would take pieces of the cancer, fly away and drop them way far away. Wherever the doves would drop the pieces, the pieces would do something good for someone somewhere. It was something I was 'playing' with. It was an experiment. But for the first time in a very long time, I had time to think. To experiment. I was taking the time to train myself to think more positively with no outside influence of what was the right thing to do or the wrong thing to do. There were no doctors or nurses calling to tell me I *had* to do it their way. The last thing I wanted to be thinking about when I was trying to think positively was that the doctors kept saying I would die if I failed to follow their suggestions.

Part of me thought, they are doctors, they know about stuff like this, they could be right. But a bigger part of me thought, I'm smart. I live in this body. There is a huge possibility that my way is right too. I just knew I wasn't going to die. And I *knew* the cancer was going to go away. It seemed there was nothing else I *could* think.

If I would have focused on the idea of the cancer growing each day, that may have been the end of me. I believe if you think cancer is going to grow, then it will grow. It's almost like giving it permission to grow. The more you pay attention to the cancer, the more you focus on it, the more powerful it becomes. I was against giving it more power. I was pouring love onto it, into it, around it. Pouring on as much love as I could imagine. Everything I was doing was based on the idea of love being involved in some way.

I believed the cancer was there, but that it could be gone. Or if it stayed it couldn't hurt me. And if it left me, it wouldn't go on to hurt anyone else. I believed if I loved whatever cancer was there, the part that was staying; if I loved it enough, it would change the cancer to some other *thing*. That it might be *like* cancer, but couldn't do any harm. It was a two-fold visualization. The love I visualized was just a word, the letters L-O-V-E. White letters. But it was nearing the end of May and I was getting better at dealing with this cancer thing.

June 1990

I can see now there were a lot of have-tos in my life. I can see now that I bought into that kind of thinking. I followed a lot of rules people put in place for me. By society, by family, by government. I had believed for a long time there were a lot of things I was supposed to do. And then one day I thought, really? Are those things going to keep me alive? Do those things have anything to do with keeping me alive? If I do my hair a certain way and wear these fashionable clothes and listen to this kind of popular music or that kind of music, is that really going to keep me alive? If I clean the bathroom on Tuesdays or arrange my spices alphabetically will that help? So I switched my thinking to do what my gut said, what my heart said. I listened to the birds and the trees. It might seem cliché, but when I started to listen to my heart I started to get well.

> It didn't take long to get rid of the cancer.

It didn't take long to get rid of the cancer. I was diagnosed in February, and by May I was starting to feel better. By June I was pretty much starting to feel like my old self. I just needed a little more time, and I figured I'd be good as new. I could feel my energy coming back, the kind of energy I was used to.

About the middle of June I moved my freezer out of the basement of the old place where Jim was living and brought it over to the motel. I moved it by myself by tying it to the truck and pulling it up some ramps on the stairs. I was stronger by then, and was feeling up to getting more of my things over to the new place. I have always prided myself on being strong for my size. I've always been on the small side and it has always been important for me to be strong, or at least *feel* strong.

> I've taught myself to figure out ways to do things on my own because I've just had to do that all my life.

I've taught myself to figure out ways to do things on my own because I've just had to do that all my life. I figure out ways to move heavy things without bugging anybody else. And I learn a lot when I have to do things like that. I'm not that strong anymore, so I really have to think harder now how to do it without hurting myself or taking up too much time. I've still got my wits about me in that area.

I stayed living in the motel room for a year. When I was feeling better I built a small chicken coop. And when I was feeling even better, I decided to tackle building a house on the property. If I could build a chicken coop, I figured I could build a house. That was in 1992.

I think if cancer seems to come as a surprise to someone, then they must have thought of getting cancer somewhere along the line. They had a fear of it. Fear enters the weakest part of a person's being, and if the fear is in their thoughts, it will enter through that avenue. From somewhere, from some little minute place, they might have thought about it, or heard about cancer, and they think they will get it, and sure enough, cancer shows up. Okay, there you go. You put that fear on it. If you could have loved it, if you could say you love it…but who is going to say something like that about cancer? Saying you love cancer goes against everything we've been taught about cancer. But what about loving your enemies?" Cancer could be the biggest enemy someone will ever face.

> Cancer could be the biggest enemy someone will ever face.

But in the Bible it says, "I say unto you, love your enemies..." (Matthew 5:44) But here's the thing. Saying you love the cancer, it changes it. The cancer changes into something else that will cause no harm. Even if you could only admit you could love it better if it wasn't cancer. If that's the best you can do, at least it's a start. I finally realized I had carried that fear all those years about my young friend dying of cancer. I met her in 1948. I remembered being so afraid that what happened to my friend would someday happen to me. After the time alone at the motel, and studying how I'd thought about things for so long, I realized being diagnosed with cancer was really no surprise to me. It was a hard truth to face. It had been a part of my thinking for so long, it's just that it was a part of me in a negative way instead of a positive one.

Someone asked me once how I learned to deal with a diagnosis like cancer. I had to think about this a bit before I could answer it in a way that made sense to me. I think it started when I was young, when I was working on my family's farm.

I learned to deal with different types of weather all my life. I believe learning ways to deal with different types of weather was a big help to me. God knew I was afraid of cancer but he also gave me the right tools and the right skills to deal with it. My job was to realize I already knew what to do. Kind of like Dorothy and her ruby slippers in the *Wizard of Oz*. I knew there was no way to change the weather, so I had to learn different ways to deal with it. I began to apply that kind of thinking so I could change what I was doing when the cancer came. I asked myself, how could I adapt? What do I need to know that I don't know? Who can I talk to who knows about cancer, especially when it comes to surviving a cancer diagnosis? What do I already know that I can apply to fixing this, changing this? I began to search for those answers. I found the answers and then did those things.

I began writing things down, keeping simple records of my new way of thinking. Years later, I even wrote a poem about the cancer situation. My daughter interviewed me and wrote an award-winning story based on my interview. She titled it "Maxine" and entered it in the Wisconsin Regional Writers Association article category of the Jade Ring contest where it won first place in 2005.

***These are some of the thoughts I started incorporating
into my new way of thinking.***

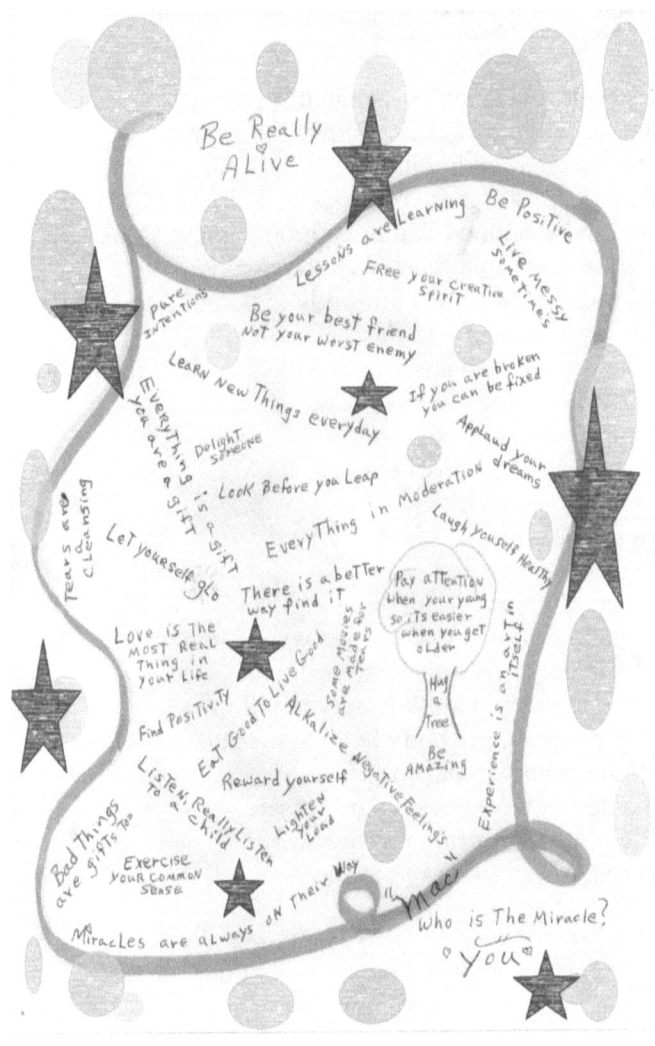

After the Cancer

This is the poem I wrote about cancer.

Finding a Better Way

By Maxine Jannette © 2007

It's been seventeen years ago this year
Doctor told me your life is over my dear
The cancer is taking its toll
It's eating right into your soul
But the Irish blood that runs through these veins
Said no, defy that fearful doctor's gains
Six months they gave this body to doom
But it wasn't about to die that soon
The doctor called almost everyday
To them I could not stray
I searched and pried
In every health book I spied
Came up with a plan
On pH balance I'd stand
I juiced and applied
Things I'd never tried
Strength returned to cells that were doomed
I could not let in no negative gloom
I'm here today with that story to tell
To the cancer, my body I would not sell
All the beauty in our life
Should not be canceled out by strife
Life is too beautiful to throw away
I found a way to make me stay.

My life has had its share of ups and down. This is the article my daughter wrote after she interviewed me fifteen years later. The cancer had not returned.

Maxine

By Julie C. Eger © 2005 (WRWA Winning Article)

I turned onto a dead end road, passed a sign that said BLESS LOVE, and slowed down as two collies came to greet me at the end of the driveway. I saw her sitting on the steps pulling a brush through her waist-length hair as I drove up to the house. I watched her clean out the brush, and hold up the long hairs. "There's more gray than I like to think about," her twinkling blue eyes smiled at me as she let the wind blow the hair from her fingers. "The birds like my hair. It helps them make very strong nests. They mix it with Casey's horsetail hair. I've found a few of the nests and they're beautiful, woven with gray, black, and a little bit of blonde."

Her name is Maxine, but most people know her as Lil' Mac. She has been a part of my life as far back as I can remember. This was so typical of her. She always had something to offer, hardly keeping anything for herself, even her own hair. She told me once that you get back what you give. I had told her I believed her reward was going to be tremendous, and she answered, "Oh, you don't think of it like that. You don't think about what you're going to get, because if it isn't what you expect, then you'll be disappointed. Just take what comes and honor it all, even the bad stuff. The most important lessons seem to be learned when the bad stuff shows up."

I had told her I wanted to interview her, it was for a class, and we were to pick someone we respected and ask them about a pivotal point in their life. She didn't question why I chose her as the person I respected.

"A pivotal point in what regard?" she asked back.

"What makes you who you are? Is there a thing that changed you, a moment when you came to believe certain things?"

"Oh, it would be hard to pick just one. Can I pick three? I can think of three things right off the bat. But let's walk through the garden while we talk. I really need to get those onions weeded."

We crossed a knee high fence and stepped into a beautifully tilled garden. We wandered past rhubarb, raspberries, strawberries and asparagus. We poked our fingers in the dirt next to corn, peas, beans, and radishes that were just popping through the fertile soil. We had to stop and look at her little patch of starter plants. "Oh look, the tomatoes are just about ready to transplant. These are supposed to be cabbages, but they don't look like cabbages. And this dill, it just grows everywhere!"

We came to the onions that were planted in long even rows. "Look, a petunia," I told her as I pointed toward a small green flower that was about ready to bloom. "Did it grow here all by itself?"

She laughed. "Oh, I suppose it could, but that's one of those little things I like to do. When I was a little girl I heard a song about someone planting a petunia in an onion patch, and ever since I've had my own garden, I've always planted one little petunia in with my onions. It makes me smile when I see it," she said as she bent to pull a stubborn weed.

"So tell me about the three things that changed your life," I asked.

"The first thing would have to be when I had my stroke. Up until then I had just taken for granted the fact that I was always fixing things. People would bring things to me and I would fix them. They would bring birds with broken wings, rabbits with broken legs, cats with broken backs, and friends with broken hearts. I don't know how I knew, but I knew how to fix them. And people kept bringing broken things. Then I learned to douse for water with a willow stick. I got very good at it. I could mark the best spots for people's wells, and even got to where I could mark how deep they would have to drill for water. Then when I was 40, I had a stroke."

"How did that change you?"

"The day I had my stroke my life changed forever. After it was over and I recovered, I didn't feel like myself anymore. Something had changed, and my ability to fix things became more pronounced. I had been searching for what it meant, this healing thing I knew about, but after the stroke it was like it had grown stronger. I know it had been there all along; but I think the stroke jarred something inside my head that made me more aware of what to do to get well. I don't know. But it was a pivotal point in my life."

"That's a pretty pivotal point. What was the second thing?"

The second thing was when I got cancer in 1990. I knew then that I had more to learn about healing. I did okay because I'm still here to talk about it, but I learned new ways to think about illnesses. The power of the mind is absolutely amazing when it comes to healing. Fear is paralyzing, and when you first learn you have an illness, it can paralyze you. When something like that happens it's important to look for the love inside yourself. Love is healing and it reflects back to you, the more love you give, the more you get back. Finding the light is essential. Keeping focused on the positive is a must. Even going beyond thinking *you will be well* to thinking *you already are well.* That was the most important lesson.

I also learned that I'm a very private person, and I had to hide to get well. Some people need the support of other people, to hold benefits for them and to pray for them. I needed to be alone so I could think about how to get myself well. I needed to be in a place where there were no distractions. I was surprised how deep I had to go to find the real love inside myself, not just the surface love I had been giving away, but the love I had for me. I had to learn to really love myself in order to get well. The more you love yourself, the more love you have to give.

I also learned that it's important to identify what you need to get well, and if you need a support system, you better get it. If you need to be alone, you better have a very good place to hide!" she smiled.

"I can't imagine what could top those two pivotal points, but tell me, what's the third one?"

"One day I was standing in my garden, after my grandkids were all grown and gone, and I realized how much I missed children. I looked up at the sky, and asked God if he couldn't find a way to bring children back into my life. Well, I guess I should have been more specific because now I'm 65 years old, and two years ago I adopted two little boys. I had them for four years before the adoption took place while the courts were trying to decide what to do. They have the same mother, but each has a different father. The courts had to give the mother and both fathers a chance to sign off as parents. Then the boys were to go up for adoption, and even though the state would do all they could to prevent it, they would separate the boys if it came to the point where they could place one but not the other. The other would stay in a foster home."

She looked at me as she placed a handful of weeds at the end of the row. "I couldn't bear having them separated. They had been together from the start. I decided to apply for the adoption even though Jim and I are so old. We had to pass all the requirements for the adoption agency, and amazingly, we were accepted. The boys are now six and eight, and doing well in school. I have so many children in my life, three children from when I was young, five grandchildren, and even two great-grandchildren. Now I have two more sons. I can't believe I'm a mom all over again," she said as a little barefoot boy ran out of the house, jumped the fence, and landed in the garden with a thud.

He came and hugged me hard around the legs. "Hi!" he said, and then took off down the onion row, his little bare feet hot in the garden sand. "Ow, ow, ow," he tiptoed away with a smile on his face, head low to the ground looking for beetles and bugs. "Mac, come see this one!"

"It doesn't get much better than this," she said as we headed down the row to look at the bug. "This is just one of my pivotal points," she said as she held the hand of the little blonde boy with amazing blue eyes who smiled up at her.

I left humbled, with a sense of awe for this woman, this little lonely petunia in a patch of onions, with her last words ringing in my ears as I drove away down the road. Before I left I had said, "Thank you for the wonderful interview."

And she replied, "Oh no, thank you. Just look at what you made me see today."

 C380

As it turned out, I discovered that two older people raising very young children in this day and age proved to be very challenging, but that is a whole other story.

Answering Questions for the Curious

One thing that happens quite often is people ask me how I knew the cancer was gone. My first inclination is to tell them that I could feel it was gone, or that I could feel it was leaving. I began to feel better every day. I began to get my energy back. I did not go back to the original doctors for any kind of check-up. I decided to listen to my body, and as long as I was feeling well, I saw no reason for further concern.

But about a year later I had what I thought was a bladder infection that seemed to be lingering longer than I liked. I made an appointment with a local doctor for that. While I was in for the bladder exam I had him *check* the cancer situation, and after doing whatever it is doctors do, he found I was clear of everything. The lump on my breast was about the size of a small chicken egg when he checked me. It turned out that it lingered for a long time, but that too, is now gone.

But ironically, *he* was unable to help me with the bladder infection, so I had to keep looking to get relief from that. I found something called D-Mannose that I got from a health food store, and that checked my bladder infection in no time. I believe quitting sugar (and when I say sugar, that includes ALL artificial sweeteners, too) helped immensely with my recurring bladder infections. I also find relief (if one should occur) by drinking homemade fresh parsley tea.

After the cancer became non-apparent, as I like to call it, I continued to explore the visualization techniques I had discovered. I continued a more healthy way of eating. I still grow wheatgrass and freeze it for a midwinter boost. I still buy a quarter or a half side of free-range beef. I raise my own chickens for meat and eggs. I stay active and look forward to my 238-step stroll to and from the mailbox each day the mail carrier drops off my mail. I don't eat foods that contain high fructose corn syrup, sugar, or hydrogenated oil. I recommend checking the labels of the foods you eat. Make your choices wisely. All the foods you buy are like a vote for what you want in life. The producers of foods will start to listen to what you vote for. They want your dollars and they get your dollars when you buy their products. It's how they make their money.

I try to be mindful of positive thoughts. I exercise my right to choose how I want to feel about my life and what I like to eat. I use mineral salt or Himalayan salt instead of the free pouring iodized-kind you usually find in a grocery store. I still stay away from refined foods and sugar. I eat a lot of raw, uncooked foods. I have a big garden and grow and preserve most of what I eat, not because I have to, but because I like to. I love gardening and growing things people can eat. I use no chemicals or pesticides in my garden.

Mostly, I never feel as though I'm deprived when other people around me are eating what they call *fun or normal food.* How can I feel deprived when the food I choose to eat helps to keep me alive to enjoy so many other things life has to offer? When I look at it from that perspective, it's easy to say no to foods that contain no energy even if they're made to taste so good you can't stop eating them once you start.

I still eat lots of fresh, homegrown greens and veggies. I had stopped eating so much fruit and I still don't eat much fruit. I learned to eat poached fish. Raw nuts and seeds. I wasn't afraid to eat real butter or coconut oil.

The yogurt mixture was nutritious enough to sustain me for a long time. Sometimes I ate breakfast at noon or later. Sometimes I still do.

I ate only when I was hungry. Rarely three meals a day. During a normal day for me, I would eat only two meals. I still only eat two meals a day. When I eat foods filled with nutrients I don't need as much because the food I choose is full of nutrition instead of empty calories. The food I eat is full of energy I can burn or full of nutrition that turns into energy I can burn. I seem to always have energy to burn. I cheat once in a while and have a good type of ice cream or a few caramels, but then I take a break from eating those things and give my *internal* system a chance to clean itself up.

I will continue to apply the new things I learned and search for new ways to experience health on as many levels as I can imagine. And as always, I will question everything and search for answers, even when I'm told it is hopeless or that my solutions will never work. I'm of the belief there is more to it than just the situation. The main thing is how you *feel* about it. It's the *feeling* I want to tap into, and why I feel that way. I believe a person has more control over their feelings than they realize. My grandmother Doyle always used to say, "Where there is a will, there is a way." It is an old quote from a Scottish author named Samuel Smiles. I believe Samuel and my Grandma Doyle knew what they were talking about. I will keep searching until I find ways that work for me. I hope you do too.

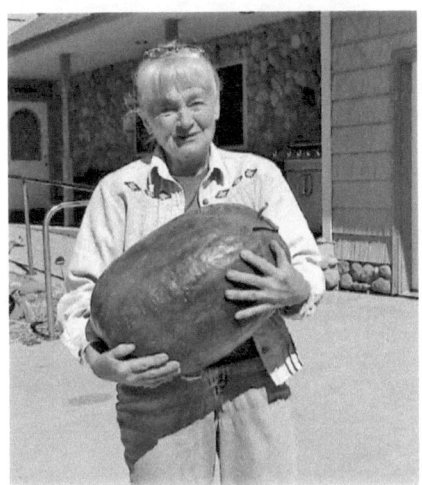

Here I am holding a 38# watermelon I grew
in my garden 22 years after the cancer.

Sept. 2011 Photo Credit: Julie C. Eger

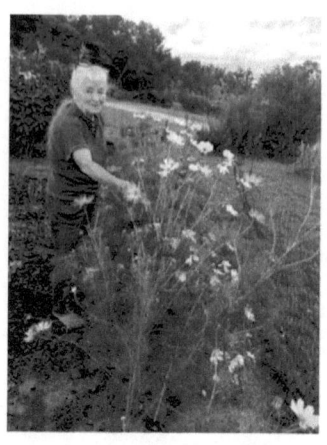

My granddaughter, Ami Mata, says she loves this picture of me. I was telling her how much I love my flowers.

October, 2014 Photo credit: Ami Mata

My Favorite Foods Now

Salad made of Tuna and Boiled Eggs

1 can organic tuna
3 chopped boiled eggs
1/2 teaspoon dry mustard
Mayonnaise to taste (no sugar in the mayo)
Salt and pepper to taste.
Eat plain, on toast or crackers.

Taco Dip Ala Maxine

16 oz. refried beans. Spread on a big platter.
8 oz. of full fat sour cream. Spread on top.
Chop a big red onion. Spread that on top.
Chop 1/2 can black olives. Spread that on top.
Chop 4 Roma tomatoes. Spread that on top.
Sprinkle 1/2 cup (or more) of salsa on top.
Sprinkle 1 cup (or more) shredded cheese on top.
(Choose your favorite cheese)
Chop Romaine lettuce for the topping. I use a lot.
Refrigerate for awhile. Use organic corn chips for
scooping up the taco dip.

Eggs for Lunch

Melt a dab of butter (the real kind) in a cast iron skillet. (I
only use cast iron and stainless steel cookware)
Add eggs. Stir to scramble. Add a bit of organic garlic salt
and a little Italian seasoning. Melt a bit of pepper jack
cheese on top.
Place the egg on a piece of toasted and buttered gluten-free
bread. Enjoy!

Bean Salad

1 can green beans or asparagus
1 can yellow beans
1 can garbanzo beans, rinsed
1 can small kidney beans, rinsed
About 8 green onions, chopped, tops and all.
About 1/4 cup or more of chopped red or green pepper.
1/2 cup apple cider vinegar
1/4 cup of olive oil
1/2 to 1 teaspoon of salt
Mix together and refrigerate.

Paprika Chicken

Melt 1 1/2 tablespoons of butter in a cast iron skillet.
1 1/2 tablespoons olive oil
2 teaspoons to 2 tablespoons chopped onion
1/2 teaspoon salt
2 teaspoons to 2 tablespoons of paprika
Cook until glossy.
Add 2 cups of organic chicken stock
Add one whole chicken, cut up.
Cover and simmer one hour.
Add 1 tablespoon of flour.
Add 1 cup of sour cream.
Serve.

Deviled Eggs

(I love these because I can grab one when I need one)
I keep deviled eggs in a glass pie pan with a glass lid so
the whole family can enjoy them. I keep them in the
refrigerator where everyone can easily grab them.
P.S. I don't make cookies!

Deviled Eggs Continued...

Six boiled eggs. Peel the eggs, cut them in half and scoop out the yolks. Place them in a bowl. Add mayonnaise, 1/2 teaspoon dry mustard, salt and pepper. Mix together and scoop back into the white halves.

Maxine Style Caviar

2 cans of black beans or black-eyed peas or 1 of each.
Drain and rinse the beans in a colander.
2 cans of white corn. Drain and rinse.
1 red pepper, chopped.
1 yellow or orange pepper, chopped.
1 green pepper, chopped.
1 to 2 jalapeno peppers, seeded, and chopped.
1 large red onion, chopped.
6 Roma tomatoes, chopped.
1 large clove of garlic, crushed
3 teaspoons of salt
2 teaspoons black pepper
1 tablespoon of hot sauce
1/2 cup balsamic vinegar
1/2 cup olive oil
1 bunch of cilantro, chopped
1/2 cup salsa
1/4 cup apple cider vinegar
1/4 cup lemon juice
Note: You may want to add more salt, balsamic vinegar, oil or whatever to match your taste). Mix and refrigerate.

How I Grew Wheat Grass

I used a ceramic plant saucer (the part that goes under a flower pot to catch the water) or a tray about 1 1/2 inches deep. Fill with potting soil and peat moss. Soak a cup of winter wheat seeds (also known as wheatberries) overnight, in a quart jar filled with warm water. Drain off the water. Let the seeds sprout for 2-3 days in the sealed jar, rinsing a couple times each day, until a small tail forms on the seed. Sprinkle the seeds on the soil. Cover with black plastic. Water the seeds each day. After 3 or 4 days, uncover the seeds and let them grow. Make sure to water them each day. When the grass starts to *split* (or grown another blade) it's time to cut your wheatgrass for juicing. Enjoy!

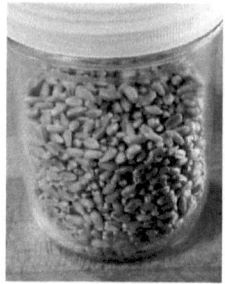

Winter wheat seeds.

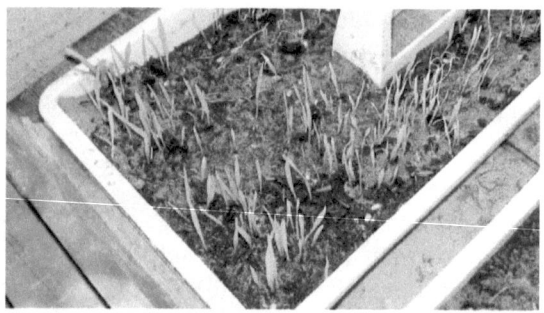

Wheatgrass as it's growing.

The End

Bibliography

Fischer, William L., **How to Fight Cancer & Win** (*Scientific guidelines and documented facts for the successful treatment and prevention of cancer and other related health problems.*) Canfield: Fischer Publishing Corporation, 1994. Print. Pgs. 66-68 Wigmore/wheatgrass, Pgs. 125, 158-160 Budwig/linseed (flax) oil theory and recipe. (*I used the original copy when I was dealing with cancer, but gave it to someone else to use, and since then have been using the 1994 revised edition.*)

Acknowledgements

I would like to thank my family and friends. You know who you are! And Michelle Desgagne (author of *The Distracted Yogi)*, Nita B. (author of *Katlyn Marie Goes For the Gold*), Eva Andrew (author of *Clutter to Calm*), Sue Wentz (author of *The Bluff, Servant to the Wolf,* and *Cassidy Creek Bridge)*, Mukulikka Ananda, and Trudi Gabryshak for all their help.

About the Author

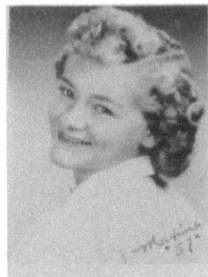

High School Graduation

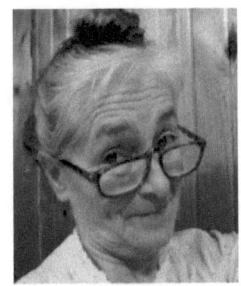

2009

My name is Maxine Jannette. At the time of this writing I am 76-years-old. I was born in Illinois, not far from the Mississippi River. I spent a lot of time on the river when I was growing up. I came to Almond, Wisconsin when I was twelve. I lived on a huge farm where we raised chickens, pigs and some cows. We also raised crops. It was hard work but I loved farming. I learned a lot and I would do it again if I could.

In 1957 I married a man whom I thought was a farmer. I had three children. It turned out my husband was better suited to carpentry and construction. I found out I loved carpentry and construction as much as I loved farming. I especially loved running the bulldozer. I've still got a lot of work to do. God isn't through with me yet!

Thank you for stopping by! I would ask a small favor that would help me out in a big way. If you enjoyed this book please take a moment to write a short review of why you enjoyed this story and post it on the site where you purchased this book. Your reviews help me to share my work with a wider audience. You can connect with my daughter on her Facebook page, **Once Upon a Blank Page,** or on my Facebook page, **Author Maxine Jannette**, for info on new releases and special promos. Remember: the kindest thing you can do for an author is to leave a kind and honest review!

Recommended reading just because my daughter, Julie C. Eger, helped me write this book and I love promoting her poems and works of fiction. Watch for the flash-fiction easy-read sequels of what happened to the characters in EENY MEENY CRIMINY CROW. Coming soon!

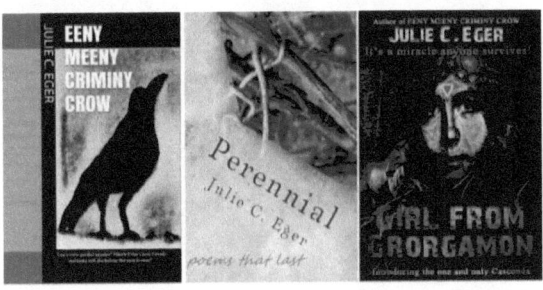

A Novel - **EENY MEENY CRIMINY CROW**

Can a crow predict murder and death?

A superstitious teenager discovers the truth from a magical lake about what happened before they caught the murdering rapist in her hometown. But will knowing the truth save the boy she loves? Will the mysterious crow's prediction about five people dying before the end of the year come true? And if so, who will survive and who will die?

Fiction/General/978-1523781140

Perennial - poems that last...

A first collection of poetry. This collection is divided into seven chapters dealing with such topics as family, relationships, religion and death. Mostly it is about survival. Falling down, getting up, and coming back better than ever. Something we can all do, a little bit, every day.

Poetry/Chapbook/978-1530316717

Girl from Grorgamon

If the taynted ones keep Casconda from avenging the Weather Master's tortured spirit it could unleash the worst weather Grorgamon Torritery has ever seen. (*Fiction/General/978-1523336517*)

About Co-Author Julie C. Eger

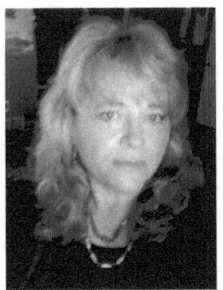

Julie lives in Wisconsin with her husband and a black Golden Doodle.

Julie has been to a few places. She's lived in houses, worn some shoes, had some hairstyles, bought a red dress, banged on drums. She knows a thing or two about rocks and totems. She's a girl, daughter, sister, woman, mother, ex-wife, wife, grandma.

She's panned for gold, water-skied over alligators in the Mississippi Bayou, spent a day at a nude beach in Jamaica. She's been in the dog house, missed a payment, burned breakfast, smelled the roses, stopped the car, stayed out too late, addressed the envelope upside down, forgot to call, ran a red light, written in the dark, sang her heart out, lived on rice and beans, slept in her car, drank too many margaritas too fast, and won a contest or two. She has loved. She has been loved. But most of all, she hopes you'll like what she's written.